Anti-Cancer Diet

Delicious Recipes for a Healthy and Balanced Lifestyle

Contents

Introduction to Cancer

Cancer is a disease that affects millions of people around the world, and is one of the leading causes of death in many countries. It is a complex condition that can start in any part of the body and affect many different types of cells. It is caused when cells divide and replicate without control, leading to the formation of a malignant tumor. Cancer can be caused by external factors or by genetic predisposition.

Cancer is divided into two main categories: malignant and benign. Malignant tumors are those that can spread to other areas of the body and are more aggressive, while benign tumors are those that can remain contained in one area. Cancer can also be classified by the type of cell it affects, such as lung cancer, breast cancer, colorectal cancer, and more.

When it comes to treatment, there are many options available. The most common treatments include surgery, radiation, chemotherapy, and immunotherapy.

Depending on the type and stage of the cancer, a combination of these treatments may be used.

It is important to remember that cancer is not a death sentence. With the help of early detection, improved treatments, and supportive care, many people are able to live with and even beat cancer. For those who are diagnosed with cancer, it is important to stay informed and to seek support from family, friends, and medical professionals.

Cancer is a difficult and challenging condition, but it does not have to be faced alone. There are many resources available to those living with cancer and their families, including support groups, information on treatments, and other helpful resources.

Cancer is a complex and difficult condition, but it can be treated and managed with the right resources and care. With the right approach, cancer can be defeated and people can live healthy, productive lives.

How Ruthie Beat Cancer

Ruthie's life changed forever when she was diagnosed with cancer. She was only 27 and had just graduated college, with big dreams for the future. But now, her dreams were put on hold as she faced a life-threatening illness.

Ruthie was determined to beat cancer, and she began researching the best treatment options available. She decided to try a combination of traditional and alternative therapies. She went through chemotherapy and radiation, but she also changed her diet, began exercising, and incorporated meditation and mindfulness into her daily routine.

Ruthie also found a strong support network of family and friends who helped her stay motivated and positive throughout her battle against cancer. She was determined to stay focused on her health, and to keep pushing forward.

After months of treatments and hard work, Ruthie finally got the news that the cancer was gone. She was overjoyed and relieved, and couldn't believe she had beaten cancer.

Ruthie had earned her victory, and she was determined to make the most of it. She used her newfound energy and resilience to pursue her dreams, and she soon found success in her career. She also opened a cancer support center, to help others who were going through the same battle she had endured.

Ruthie's story is one of courage and resilience. She was able to beat cancer and make the most of her life, and she hopes her story will inspire others to do the same.

Causes Of Cancer

Cancer is a devastating disease that affects millions of people around the world. While there is no one single cause of cancer, there are a number of factors that can increase a person's risk for developing the disease. Understanding the potential causes of cancer can help to inform prevention efforts and provide insight into potential treatments.

The first major cause of cancer is genetics. Certain genes may be passed down through families, increasing the likelihood of developing certain types of cancer. In addition, exposures to certain environmental factors, such as smoking, radiation, and certain chemicals, can increase the risk of cancer. Smoking is especially linked to lung cancer, while exposure to radiation can lead to an increased risk of developing leukemia or thyroid cancer.

Diet and lifestyle also play a role in cancer risk. Unhealthy diets high in saturated fats, processed foods, and refined sugars can increase the risk of developing certain cancers. Additionally, a lack of exercise, obesity, and excessive alcohol consumption can also increase the risk for certain types of cancer.

Infections can also cause cancer. Infections from certain viruses, such as the human papillomavirus (HPV), can cause certain types of cancer, such as cervical and anal cancer. Other viruses, such as hepatitis B and C, can lead to an increased risk of developing liver cancer.

Finally, age is a major risk factor for cancer. As people get older, their risk for developing cancer increases. This is because the body's cells become less efficient at repairing damaged DNA over time, which can lead to mutations that can lead to cancer.

Overall, cancer is a complex disease that is caused by a variety of factors, including genetics, environmental exposures, lifestyle choices, and infections. Understanding the potential causes of cancer can help to inform prevention efforts, as well as provide insight into potential treatments.

The first major cause of cancer is genetics. Certain genes may be passed down through families, increasing the likelihood of developing certain types of cancer. In addition, exposures to certain environmental factors, such as smoking, radiation, and certain chemicals, can increase the risk of cancer. Smoking is especially linked to lung cancer, while exposure to radiation can lead to an increased risk of developing leukemia or thyroid cancer.

Diet and lifestyle also play a role in cancer risk. Unhealthy diets high in saturated fats, processed foods, and refined sugars can increase the risk of developing certain cancers. Additionally, a lack of exercise, obesity, and excessive alcohol consumption can also increase the risk for certain types of cancer.

Infections can also cause cancer. Infections from certain viruses, such as the human papillomavirus (HPV), can cause certain types of cancer, such as cervical and anal cancer. Other viruses, such as hepatitis B and C, can lead to an increased risk of liver cancer.

Finally, certain medical treatments can increase the risk of developing cancer. For example, radiation therapy and chemotherapy are known to increase the risk of developing certain types of cancer.

It is important to recognize the potential causes of cancer, as this can help inform prevention efforts and potentially lead to new treatments. Genetics, lifestyle factors, infections, and medical treatments can all increase the risk of developing cancer. By understanding the potential causes of cancer, individuals can take steps to reduce their risk and possibly develop better treatments for those who are already affected.

Symptoms And Recognising Symptoms Of Cancer

Cancer can be a terrible diagnosis. It is one of the leading causes of death in the world and can affect anyone at any age. It is important to recognize the symptoms of cancer early on, as early diagnosis can make a life-saving difference.

The most common symptoms of cancer are persistent fatigue, unexplained weight loss, and pain. Other signs may include lumps or swelling, changes in skin color, or changes in bowel or bladder habits. If any of these symptoms persist for more than a few weeks, it is important to see a doctor.

In addition to these physical symptoms, psychological symptoms can also be an indication of cancer. These include feelings of helplessness, depression, anxiety, and changes in sleep patterns. If any of these symptoms are present, it is important to seek help right away.

Other signs of cancer can include a fever that does not go away, a cough that does not improve, or a sore that does not heal.

These symptoms can also be indicators of other illnesses, so it is important to have them checked out by a doctor to rule out any other possible causes.

Cancer can also cause changes in your body's metabolism. If you find yourself feeling more tired than usual, having difficulty digesting food, or having changes in your appetite, these could be signs of an underlying cancer.

It is important to be aware of any changes in your body, even if they seem minor. If any of these symptoms persist for more than a few weeks, it is important to seek medical advice. Early detection of cancer can make a life-saving difference.

Cancer can be a difficult diagnosis to receive, but it is important to remember that it is treatable and that with the right treatment, a full recovery is possible. It is important to stay informed and to recognize the symptoms of cancer, so that if you or someone you know is experiencing them, help can be sought as quickly as possible.

Diagnosis and Treatment Options of cancer

Cancer is a life-threatening disease that affects millions of people worldwide. It is a complex and devastating illness that requires specialized care and treatment. The diagnosis and treatment of cancer can vary significantly depending on the type, stage, and location of the cancer. It is important for individuals to understand the diagnosis and treatment options available to them so that they can make informed decisions about their care.

When someone is diagnosed with cancer, the physician will first need to determine the type and stage of the cancer. This is done through a variety of tests, such as blood tests, imaging studies, and biopsies. Depending on the type of cancer, the doctor may also need to assess the extent of the cancer to determine the best treatment plan.

Once the type and stage of the cancer have been determined, the doctor can begin to discuss treatment options with the patient. Treatment options can vary depending on the type and stage of the cancer, as well as the individual's overall health. Common treatments for cancer include chemotherapy, radiation therapy, surgery, and immunotherapy.

Chemotherapy is a common treatment used to kill cancer cells. This type of treatment is usually given intravenously and can involve a combination of different drugs. The drugs work by targeting and killing cancer cells while leaving healthy cells intact. Radiation therapy is another common treatment option that utilizes high-energy x-rays to kill cancer cells. Radiation therapy can be used alone or in conjunction with other treatments.

Surgery is also an option for some types of cancer. The goal of surgery is to remove the cancer and any nearby tissue that may have been affected by the cancer. In some cases, doctors may also use chemotherapy or radiation therapy before or after surgery in order to help ensure that all of the cancerous cells have been removed.

Immunotherapy is an increasingly popular treatment option for certain types of cancer. This type of therapy works by stimulating the body's own immune system to recognize and attack cancer cells. It is generally used in combination with other treatments and is often used in cases where other treatments have been unsuccessful.

No matter what type of cancer a person is diagnosed with, it is important to understand the diagnosis and treatment options available. It is also important to speak with the doctor about any potential risks or side effects associated with the various treatments. With proper care and treatment, many types of cancer can be successfully treated and managed.

Natural Remedies for Cancer

Cancer is a devastating disease that can affect anyone, regardless of age, gender, or ethnicity. Although there is no sure-fire way to prevent cancer, there are some natural remedies that may help reduce your risk of developing the disease.

One of the most important ways to reduce your risk of cancer is to maintain a healthy lifestyle. Eating a balanced diet, exercising regularly, and getting adequate rest can all help to keep your body functioning at its best. Additionally, staying away from unhealthy habits such as smoking and excessive alcohol consumption can help to minimize your chances of developing cancer.

Herbal remedies can also be effective in reducing the risk of cancer. Several herbs have been used for centuries to help with cancer-related issues. Green tea, for instance, is packed with antioxidants which help to fight free radicals, reducing the risk of developing cancer. Turmeric is another popular herb that has anti-inflammatory properties, helping to reduce inflammation in the body which can lead to cancer.

Stress can also be a major factor in the development of cancer. Taking steps to reduce stress in your life can help to reduce your risk of developing the disease. Meditation, yoga, and other relaxation techniques can help to alleviate stress and promote overall health.

In addition to these lifestyle changes, there are also a few supplements that have been linked to reducing the risk of cancer. Vitamin D is one of the most commonly used supplements, as it has been shown to reduce inflammation in the body and improve overall health. Omega-3 fatty acids are also beneficial, as they are thought to help reduce inflammation and reduce the risk of cancer.

Although there is no cure for cancer, there are natural remedies that may help to reduce your risk of developing the disease. Eating a healthy diet, exercising regularly, and reducing stress are all important steps that can help to keep your body functioning at its best. Additionally, supplements such as Vitamin D and Omega-3 fatty acids can help to reduce inflammation and improve overall health. Making these lifestyle changes can help to reduce your risk of developing cancer and increase your chances of living a long and healthy life.

Herbal Remedies for Cancer treatment

Herbal remedies have been used for centuries to treat a wide range of ailments, including cancer. While there is no cure for cancer, the use of herbal remedies to reduce symptoms and improve quality of life is becoming increasingly popular.

Herbal remedies are derived from plants and may be taken as a tea, an extract, a tincture, or in capsule or tablet form. Herbal remedies may be used in conjunction with conventional cancer treatments, such as chemotherapy and radiation, or may be used as an alternative treatment for cancer.

The use of herbal remedies for cancer treatment is controversial, as there is limited scientific evidence to support their effectiveness. However, some studies have suggested that certain herbs may have anti-cancer properties.

One of the most widely-studied herbs for cancer is turmeric. Turmeric contains curcumin, a compound that has been found to have anti-inflammatory and antioxidant properties. Studies suggest that curcumin may be beneficial for people with certain types of cancer, such as colorectal, prostate, and breast cancer.

Another herb that has been studied for its potential cancer-fighting properties is green tea. Green tea contains compounds called catechins, which are antioxidants that can help protect cells from damage caused by free radicals. Studies suggest that catechins may be beneficial for people with certain types of cancer, such as colorectal, prostate, and breast cancer.

Ginseng is another herb that may have cancer-fighting properties. Ginseng contains compounds called ginsenosides, which may have antioxidant and anti-inflammatory properties. Studies suggest that ginsenosides may help reduce the growth of cancer cells and reduce the risk of certain types of cancer.

While there is limited scientific evidence to support the use of herbal remedies for cancer treatment, some studies suggest that certain herbs may have anti-cancer properties. Before taking any herbal remedy, it is important to talk to your doctor to ensure that it is safe and appropriate for your condition.

Stress Management for cancer

As a cancer survivor, I know firsthand how difficult it can be to manage stress. In a world filled with uncertainty and fear, it can be hard to stay focused on the positive. Thankfully, there are a variety of strategies that can help us manage our stress levels, even in the face of a cancer diagnosis.

The first step in managing stress is to recognize it and identify the triggers. The American Institute of Stress recommends that people keep a journal and document their thoughts and feelings about any stressful event. This can help provide valuable insight into patterns and habits that can be addressed.

Once the triggers are identified, the next step is to develop a plan of action. This might include relaxation techniques such as deep breathing, yoga, or meditation. Exercise is also important, as it helps to reduce stress hormones in the body.

Another strategy is to establish a healthy lifestyle. Eating well, getting enough sleep, and engaging in activities such as socializing, reading, or listening to music can help to reduce stress levels.

It is also important to reach out for help when needed. Seeking the support of loved ones, friends, and professionals can be invaluable in managing stress.

Finally, it is important to remember that the journey with cancer is unique to each individual. Everyone responds differently to stress, so it is important to find what works best for you.

Managing stress can be difficult, but it is an important part of living with cancer. By recognizing the triggers, developing a plan of action, and seeking help when needed, we can better manage our stress levels and focus on the positive.

Diet and Exercise for cancer treatment

When it comes to cancer treatment, diet and exercise can play a powerful role in helping to improve the quality of life for those affected. In fact, recent studies have shown that proper nutrition and physical activity can help to reduce the risk of developing certain types of cancer.

A healthy diet is essential for cancer patients. Eating a variety of foods from all food groups is important for proper nutrition. It's important to get enough protein, carbohydrates, fats, vitamins, and minerals in order to maintain a healthy weight and provide the body with the nutrients it needs. It's also important to limit processed and sugary foods, as well as red and processed meats.

In addition to a healthy diet, regular physical activity is also important for cancer patients. Exercise can help to strengthen the body and reduce the risk of certain types of cancer. It can also help to reduce fatigue, improve mood, and reduce depression.

For cancer patients, it's important to talk to the doctor about the best type of exercise for them. Exercise should be tailored to the individual's needs and abilities. It's also important to start slowly and increase the intensity of the exercise gradually.

In addition to diet and exercise, there are other lifestyle changes that cancer patients can make to help improve their health.

These include quitting smoking, limiting alcohol intake, and getting enough sleep. All of these lifestyle changes can help to reduce the risk of cancer and improve quality of life.

Overall, diet and exercise are two important components of cancer treatment. Eating a healthy diet and getting regular physical activity can help to reduce the risk of certain types of cancer and improve quality of life for cancer patients. It's important to talk to the doctor about the best type of diet and exercise plan for the individual. With proper nutrition and physical activity, cancer patients can improve their health and quality of life. `

write a powerful and creative article on Alternative Treatments for cancer

The diagnosis of cancer is devastating for individuals and their families. Conventional treatments for cancer, such as surgery, radiation, and chemotherapy, are often harsh and debilitating. Fortunately, there are many alternative treatments for cancer that have been proven to be just as effective in treating the disease as conventional treatments.

One of the most popular alternative treatments for cancer is herbal medicine. Herbal medicine is a form of alternative medicine that uses plants and plant extracts to treat various ailments. Many herbs have been found to possess anti-cancer properties and can be used to treat various types of cancer. Examples of herbs that may be used to treat cancer include turmeric, ginger, green tea, garlic, and licorice root.

Another popular alternative treatment for cancer is acupuncture. Acupuncture is a form of Traditional Chinese Medicine that involves inserting thin needles into specific points on the body. Studies have shown that acupuncture can reduce pain and symptoms associated with cancer, as well as improve quality of life.

Cannabis is another alternative treatment for cancer that has been gaining popularity in recent years. Cannabis has been found to contain numerous anti-cancer properties and has been found to be effective in treating many types of cancer. Cannabis has also been found to reduce pain, nausea, and other side effects associated with cancer treatments.

Diet and nutrition are also important when it comes to treating cancer. Eating a healthy diet full of fruits, vegetables, and lean proteins can help to boost the body's natural defenses and improve overall health. Eating a diet that is low in fat and processed foods can also help to reduce the risk of cancer.

Lastly, exercise is another important alternative treatment for cancer. Regular exercise can help to boost the immune system and reduce stress levels. Exercise can also help to reduce fatigue and improve overall quality of life.

Alternative treatments for cancer are becoming increasingly popular as more and more people look for ways to treat their disease without having to undergo harsh and debilitating conventional treatments. While not all alternative treatments are effective in treating cancer, many have been found to be just as effective as conventional treatments. It is important to speak to your doctor before beginning any alternative treatment to ensure it is safe and effective for you.

Acupuncture for cancer treatment

Acupuncture, an ancient Chinese practice, has been used for centuries to treat a variety of ailments. Recently, researchers have begun to explore the use of acupuncture for cancer treatment. The idea of using needles to stimulate the body's healing processes has been gaining traction as an alternative form of cancer therapy.

Acupuncture involves inserting thin needles into specific points on the body to stimulate various areas of the body and to balance energy. In traditional Chinese medicine, unbalanced energy is thought to be the source of many diseases, including cancer. By restoring balance to the body's energy, acupuncture may be able to help the body heal itself and fight off cancer.

There is a growing body of research that supports the use of acupuncture for cancer treatment. Studies have shown that acupuncture can help reduce symptoms such as nausea and pain associated with chemotherapy and radiation. It can also improve quality of life by reducing stress and anxiety.

In addition, acupuncture may have direct anti-cancer effects. Studies have found that acupuncture can help boost the immune system and reduce inflammation, both of which can help the body fight off cancer. Acupuncture can also reduce the side effects of chemotherapy and radiation, allowing patients to receive more effective treatments.

Despite the promising research, it's important to remember that acupuncture is not a replacement for conventional cancer treatments. It should be used in conjunction with traditional treatments such as chemotherapy and radiation. It can be a valuable tool for symptom relief and for improving overall quality of life during cancer treatment, however.

Acupuncture is a safe and effective way to manage the side effects of cancer treatment and improve overall quality of life. While more research is needed to fully understand the benefits of acupuncture for cancer treatment, the current evidence suggests that it can be a powerful tool in the fight against cancer.

Holistic Approach

The benefits of a holistic approach to health and wellness are plentiful and far-reaching. Holistic health is an approach to health that focuses on the whole person – their physical, mental, emotional and spiritual health – rather than just one aspect of their existence. It emphasizes the importance of connecting with the body, mind and spirit to achieve optimal health and wellness.

The holistic approach is based on the idea that the body has a natural ability to heal itself when given the right environment, nutrition and lifestyle choices. It takes into account the individual's overall health and lifestyle, as well as their personal preferences. Holistic health focuses on prevention, rather than just treating symptoms. By taking a holistic approach to health, individuals can identify potential health issues before they become serious, and make changes to their lifestyle to prevent them from occurring.

One of the main benefits of the holistic approach to health is that it takes into account the individual's physical, mental, and spiritual health. This means that individuals can address all aspects of their wellbeing, rather than just focusing on one area. For example, someone dealing with depression can benefit from a holistic approach to health, as it would involve exploring the underlying causes of their depression, as well as addressing their physical and mental health.

The holistic approach also recognizes the importance of personalizing health and wellness plans. Rather than following a one-size-fits-all approach, a holistic health plan takes into account the individual's unique needs and preferences, and creates a plan that is tailored to them. This ensures that individuals are working on a plan that is tailored to their specific needs and preferences, rather than one that may not work for them.

Finally, the holistic approach to health and wellness allows individuals to take control of their own health, rather than relying on medical professionals to do it for them. By taking a holistic approach to health, individuals can learn how to make lifestyle changes that will benefit their overall health and wellbeing. This can include learning how to manage stress, eating a balanced diet, getting enough sleep, and making time for exercise.

In summary, the holistic approach to health and wellness offers numerous benefits. It emphasizes the importance of addressing the physical, mental, and spiritual aspects of health, as well as taking into account the individual's unique needs and preferences. It also allows individuals to take control of their own health, rather than relying on medical professionals to do it for them. With the right lifestyle changes, individuals can achieve optimal health and wellbeing.

Benefits of acupuncture

Acupuncture is an ancient form of therapy that dates back thousands of years and has been used in many cultures to treat a variety of ailments. In recent years, acupuncture has gained popularity in the United States due to its effectiveness in treating a wide range of conditions. Acupuncture is a holistic, non-invasive form of natural healing that works to stimulate the body's own healing abilities. By inserting fine needles into specific points on the body, acupuncture can help to restore balance and harmony to the body's various systems.

The benefits of acupuncture are numerous and varied. It can be used to treat a wide range of physical, mental, and emotional conditions. Acupuncture is known to reduce pain, improve sleep, and improve digestion. It can also help to reduce stress, improve mood, and increase energy levels. Additionally, acupuncture can be used to treat conditions such as headaches, allergies, asthma, arthritis, and muscle tension.

In addition to its physical and emotional benefits, acupuncture has also been found to have numerous physiological benefits. Acupuncture can help to regulate the body's hormones, boost the immune system, and increase circulation. It can also improve the body's ability to absorb nutrients, improve organ function, and promote healing. Acupuncture can even be used to improve fertility and reduce the risk of some types of cancer.

Finally, acupuncture can also provide psychological benefits. It can help to reduce anxiety, improve self-esteem, and improve concentration. Additionally, acupuncture can be used to reduce the symptoms of depression and anxiety, and even help to reduce the risk of relapse for those with substance abuse issues.

Overall, acupuncture is a powerful and safe form of natural healing with numerous benefits. It can be used to treat a wide range of physical, mental, and emotional conditions. Additionally, it has numerous physiological and psychological benefits. For anyone looking for a natural way to improve their health and wellness, acupuncture is definitely worth considering.

Coping with Side Effects of cancer treatment

Cancer is a devastating disease that can be physically and emotionally draining. The treatments and medications used to fight cancer can be extremely effective, but they can also have side effects that can make the process even more difficult. Coping with the side effects of cancer treatment can be challenging, but there are several strategies that can help.

The first step in coping with the side effects of cancer treatment is to understand what to expect. Treatment side effects vary depending on the type of cancer and the type of treatment being used. Common side effects can include fatigue, nausea, hair loss, skin changes, and cognitive changes. Learning about what to expect from the treatment can help individuals prepare and manage their expectations.

The second step is to talk to a doctor or health care provider. Health care providers can provide information on how to best manage side effects and can also provide helpful resources such as support groups, counseling, and dietary recommendations. Talking to a doctor or health care provider can also help individuals determine if there are any medications or treatments that can help with the side effects.

The third step is to practice self-care. Self-care is an important part of managing side effects and can include activities such as exercise, relaxation, and eating a healthy diet. Exercise, in particular, can help to reduce fatigue, improve mood, and boost energy levels. Additionally, getting enough rest and avoiding stressful situations can also help to manage side effects.

The fourth step is to reach out for support. Cancer can be an isolating experience, so it is important to seek out support from friends, family, and other cancer survivors. Support groups can provide a safe space to talk about the side effects of treatment, share experiences, and get practical advice on managing side effects.

Finally, it is important to take time for yourself. Cancer treatment can be an all-consuming process, so it is important to take time to do things that bring joy and pleasure. This can include activities such as reading, listening to music, going for walks, or spending time with friends and family.

Coping with the side effects of cancer treatment can be difficult, but there are ways to manage them. By understanding the side effects, talking to a doctor or health care provider, practicing self-care, reaching out for support, and taking time for yourself, individuals can better cope with the side effects of cancer treatment.

10 Ways Fight Off Cancer

The Best Tips On How To Keep This Killer At Bay

Synopsis

According to the National Cancer Institute, roughly 1/3 of all cancer deaths may be ascribed to our diets. The advocated diet isn't elaborate or expensive. There are a lot of foods and even spices that may very well help in the fight against cancer. Some authorities claims that a lot of healthy food choices will help reduce the possibility of contracting cancer, and may shrivel up tumors.

Eat Right

There are a lot of factors that put up contribute to cancer. According to Mayo Clinic, inadequate diet, obesity and smoking give the sack cause cancer. Genetic endowment is likewise a factor in some forms of cancer. It's simple enough to protect yourself from skin cancer. You should utilize sunscreen during the daylight hours to protect your skin from UV rays

Cruciferous veggies like broccoli, cauliflower, kale, brussel sprouts and cabbage hold 2 major antioxidants-lutein and zeanthin. These antioxidants might help battle against prostate cancer. Most of the fresh veggies in the food market contain antioxidants, vitamins and minerals, which might aid in the prevention of cancer.

Oranges and lemons perk up the immune system to drive back cancer cells. Papayas bear ascorbic acid, which works as an antioxidant. Raspberries hold a lot of vitamins and minerals which help protect against cancer. Nuts hold a lot of antioxidants, which might suppress the growth of tumors.

Some authorities explain that tea is determined to have cancer-fighting powers. While all teas are good for the body, green tea is made from unfermented tea leaves. Consequently, it has the highest density of antioxidants. The antioxidants in tea are known as polyphenols.

An article issued in 2007 by the University of Maryland Medical Center explicates that polyphenols are thought to battle free radicals. Although free radicals come about naturally in the body, they're believed to be the leading cause of many diseases, including cancer. The polyphenols in green tea might counterbalance these free radicals, and might even reduce or prevent harm to the body.

According to some authorities, garlic bears allum compounds that seem to support the immune system. Turmeric, which is a member of the ginger family, likewise helps battle cancer. Hot chile peppers and jalapenos bear capsaicin, which is thought to be a cancer fighting agent. Rosemary, which is a flavorful spice, might help in the battle against cancer.

Synopsis

Fresh research affirms what nutritionists have stated for years: consuming lots of high-fiber foods is a capital way to protect your health. That may sound like a steep claim. But according to investigators conducting the biggest-ever study into the relationship between diet and cancer, it's the facts.

Use Fiber

Some may feel the jury is still out on fiber's role as a cancer fighter. All the same, given the many advantages of high-fiber foods like whole grains, fruits, and veggies, the arguments for contributing more fiber to your diet are overpowering. A high-fiber diet may cut levels of blood cholesterol, help keep up regularity, and avert gastrointestinal conditions like diverticulitis.

Contrary to their processed counterparts, like white rice or white bread, whole-grain foods hold their original fiber, the nutrient-rich bran and germ, and the starchy endosperm. That may sound academic, but from a nutritional point of view it makes a huge difference.

Processing whole grains to produce a refined grain takes away most of their nutritional content. Individuals erroneously believe that the laws calling for white flour to be enriched counterbalance for the many useful nutrients lost during processing. It's straight that a few synthetic vitamins and minerals are added to our white flour, but this does not even come close to reestablishing all the lost nutrients.

Whole wheat, for instance, contains calcium, iron, magnesium, phosphorus, sodium, zinc, copper, manganese, and selenium. It likewise has vitamin C, thiamin, riboflavin, niacin, pantothen, vitamin B6, folate, and vitamin E.

The body changes all carbohydrates into glucose. But it breaks down processed grains much faster than intact grains. The speedy breakdown of processed carbs often causes wide sways in blood glucose that may trigger hunger cravings, cause the release of tension hormones, and originate the buildup of arterial plaques.

Basic whole grains include brown rice, barley, millet, oats, buckwheat, rye, and whole wheat. You may also want to try out some traditional Native American grains such as quinoa ("keen-wa") or amaranth, found in health-food stores. Good whole-grain recipes are simple to discover on the net. But savoring these highly nutritious foods may require patience-whole grains commonly take longer to cook than refined grains.

Synopsis

Toxins and Pollutants are brought into our homes day-after-day through water, food, dirt, dust and household cleansing products. For instance, the serious toxin phenol may be detected in a few disinfectants, antiseptics and even air fresheners. Continued exposure to phenols and additional toxins might have injurious effects on our nervous and respiratory systems, also induce cancers. It's crucial to educate yourself to enable you to cut down your risk and exposure. When you start to educate yourself about the chemicals and toxins on the labels of the products in your house, you might prefer to substitute some of the toxic agents you discover with non-toxic options.

No Toxins

Cautiously read the list of components on all labels of your household products to make certain you're not utilizing products that contains adverse toxins. If you check out http://www.leas.ca/Cleaners-and-Toxins.htm and click on the cleaners and toxins, it will take you to a really enlightening site and you'll be able to download this data. You'll learn about a lot of risky substances, one of them being Silica that's detected in many abrasive cleansers, and about a powerful reproductive toxin Toluene [which is in many nail polishes].

Pick your seafood with wisdom in order to limit the measure of mercury that you absorb. Restrict the amount of canned tuna fish and avoid swordfish, shark, and bluefish and rather buy wild salmon, tilapia or Pacific cod. Prevent frying food and utilize grilling, broiling or roasting cooking techniques. If possible buy organic when selecting those fruits and veggies that otherwise have the highest pesticide levels.

Set up a water filter to prevent the consumption of heavy metals. You are able to review the performance rating of a lot of top brands of water filters by Googling water filter comparisons, where there are a lot of sites to choose from.

Attempt to minimize the utilization of Teflon or any additional pan that has a non-stick coating. The Environmental Working Group discovered that this cookware more rapidly reaches temperatures that bring about toxic particles and fumes. You might want to pick stainless steel or cast iron for your cookware.

Never microwave in plastic. Utilize packaging that's labeled "microwave safe" or utilize glass or ceramic containers. Although the literature is controversial, many health advocacy groups feel that dioxin is brought out in plastic when its micro waved.

Be conservative about utilizing antibacterial soaps. They may contain pesticides that may be absorbed through the skin and aren't healthy for the environment. Utilize a simple soap with water and scrub hands for twenty seconds.

Attempt to minimize the utilization of herbicides and insecticides. The toxic components can get into our system by skin contact and inhalation.

Take off your shoes before walking into the house. Pesticides from outdoor dust, lawns and invisible toxins on the ground may be easily tracked from outdoors back into your house and persist there for long periods.

Restrict your use of bleach and utilize lemon juice alternatively for whitening. Just because a few companies are getting great "green marketing gimmicks" don't trust the advertising. Read all components on your detergent bottles. Restrict the amount of chemicals mixing with your clothes by averting the addition of any softeners into your washer or dryer.

If you get any of your clothing cleaned from pro cleaners, let these clothing items remain outside for about eight hours to keep some of the chemicals and odors from returning into your house.

Forever vacuum with a filter or even more beneficial a HEPA filter. A HEPA filter snares very small particles that other vacuums might re-circulate back into the air of your house. Since there may be multiple allergens in your house, including dust mites, vacuum and dust on a regular basis.

Pick your personal products and cosmetics that are created by companies that don't have toxic elements. You are able to look up products on the web that you either are presently using or research data on products you're considering buying for known or suspected hazards. Although a product might be listed as low hazard on a site, there's no guarantee that it's safe. You likewise need to check on the safety of the products listed in the low hazard groups.

www.ingramcontent.com/pod-product-compliance
Lightning Source LLC
Chambersburg PA
CBHW061603250726
48657CB00017B/1798